T0198971

LIFE
IS STILL
Sweet

My Sibling has Type 1 Diabetes

Written by Jennifer Bracci

Illustrated by Angie Jones

Balboa Press books may be ordered through booksellers or by contacting:

Balboa Press
A Division of Hay House
1663 Liberty Drive
Bloomington, IN 47403
www.balboapress.com
844-682-1282

ISBN: 979-8-7652-3193-7 (sc)
ISBN: 979-8-7652-3194-4 (e)

Library of Congress Control Number: 2022913995

Print information available on the last page.

Balboa Press rev. date: 02/24/2023

BALBOA.PRESS

For Dillon, Patrick and Emma -JB
For Don, Kyle, Lillie and Ralyn -AJ

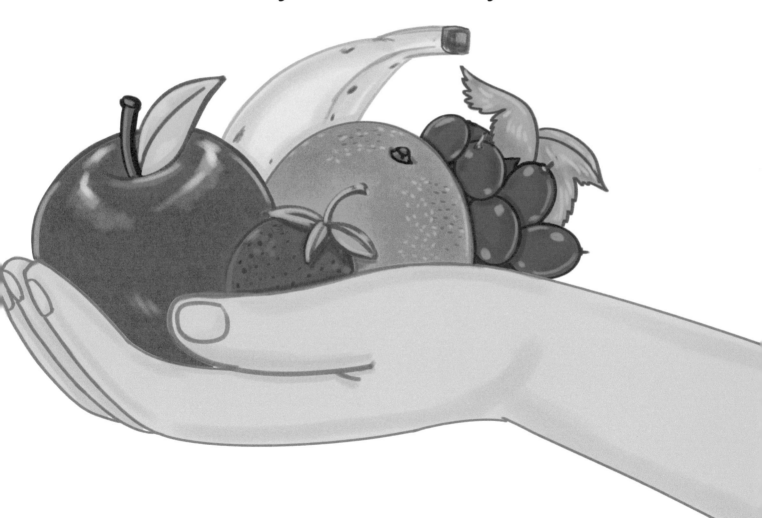

There's a party next week for my best friend. I know I will not want that day to end.

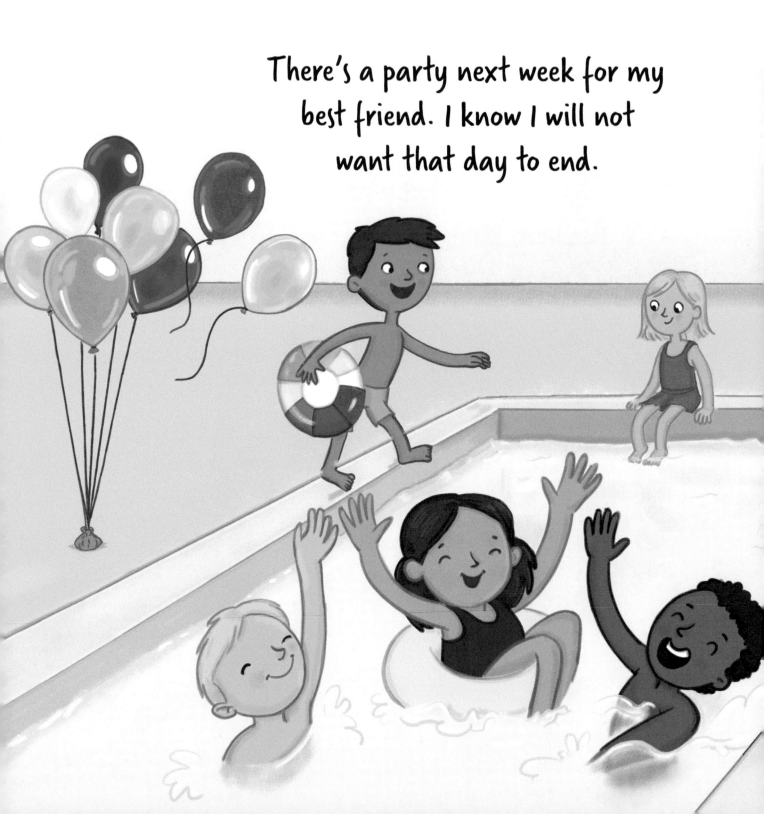

This party has me in such a great mood. Swimming, balloons and a whole lot of food.

Cookies and cupcakes with frosting so sweet!

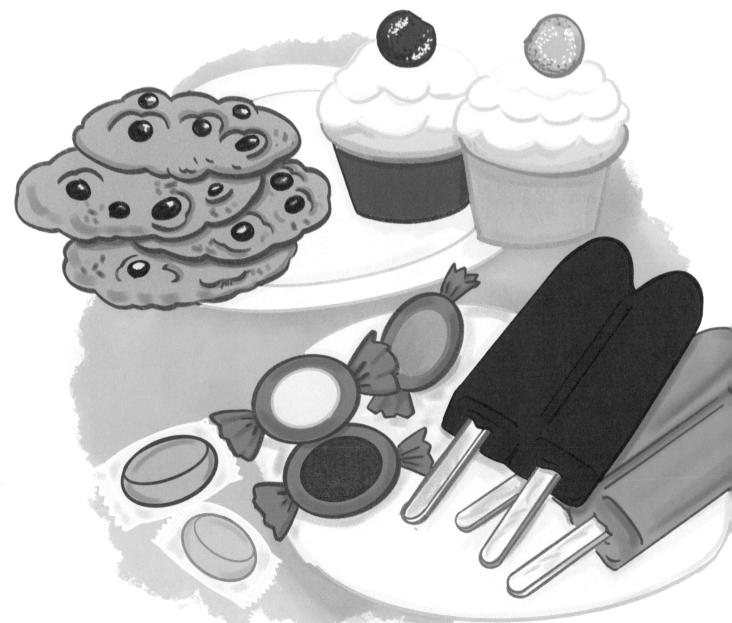

Candy and popsicles! What a good treat!

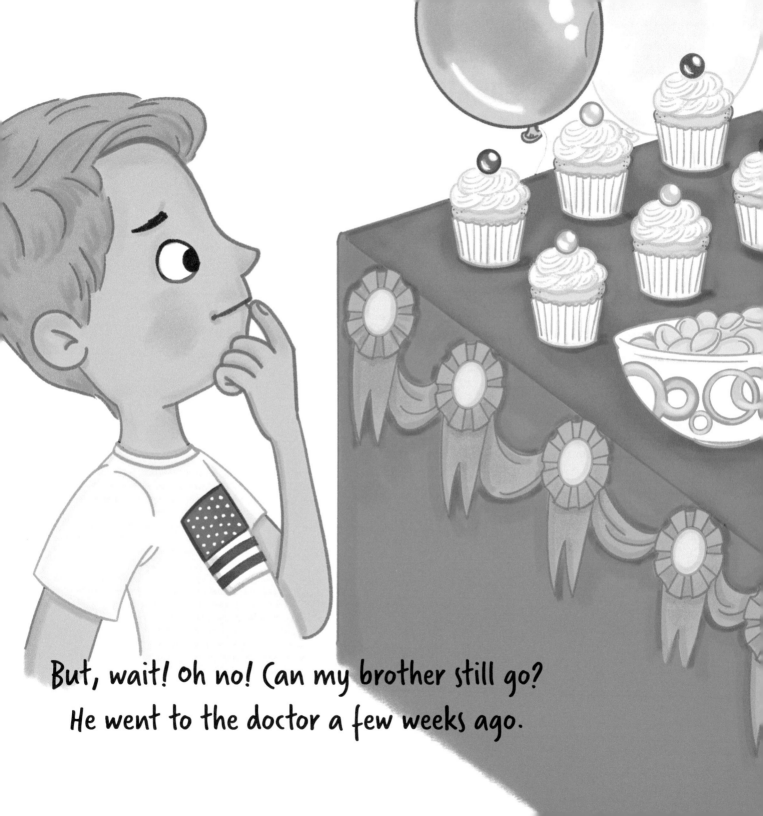

But, wait! oh no! Can my brother still go?
He went to the doctor a few weeks ago.

We always ate healthy. How could this be?
We ran outdoors. He was faster than me.

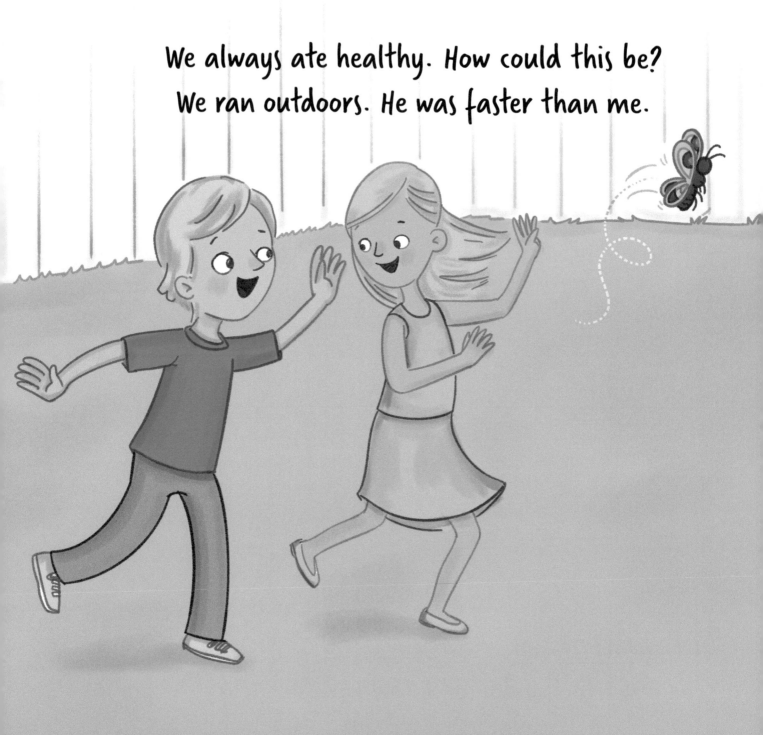

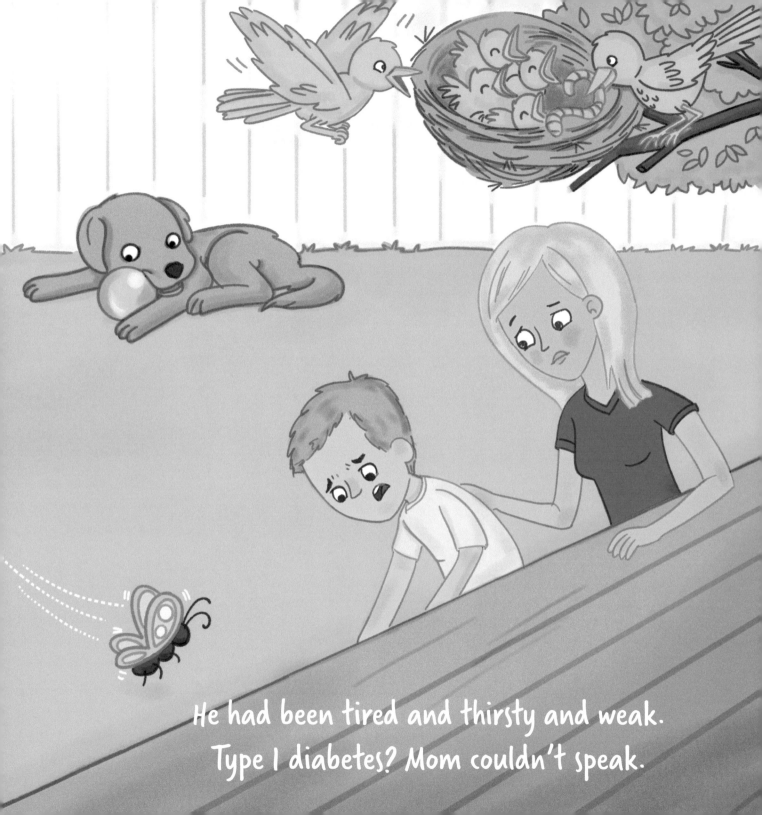

He had been tired and thirsty and weak.
Type 1 diabetes? Mom couldn't speak.

How did this happen? Dad wanted to know.
Doctors must teach us before we could go.

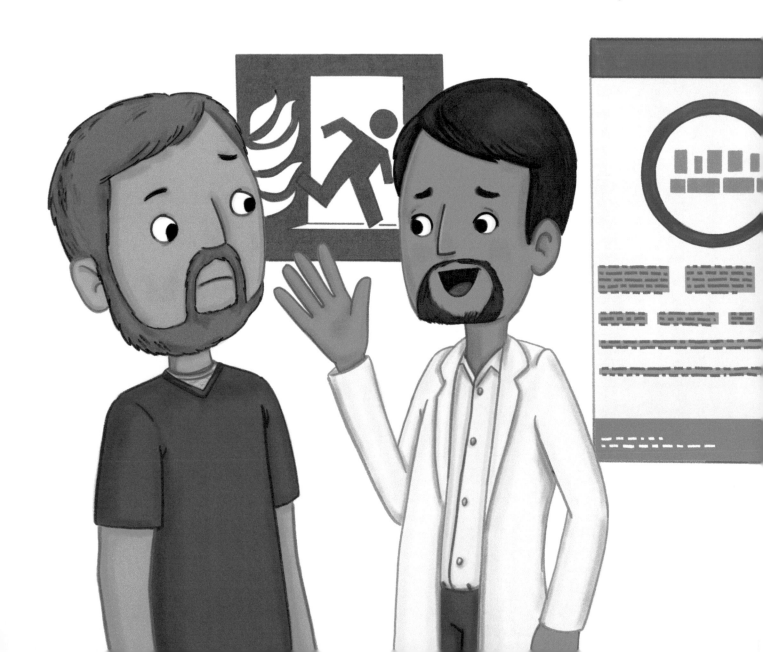

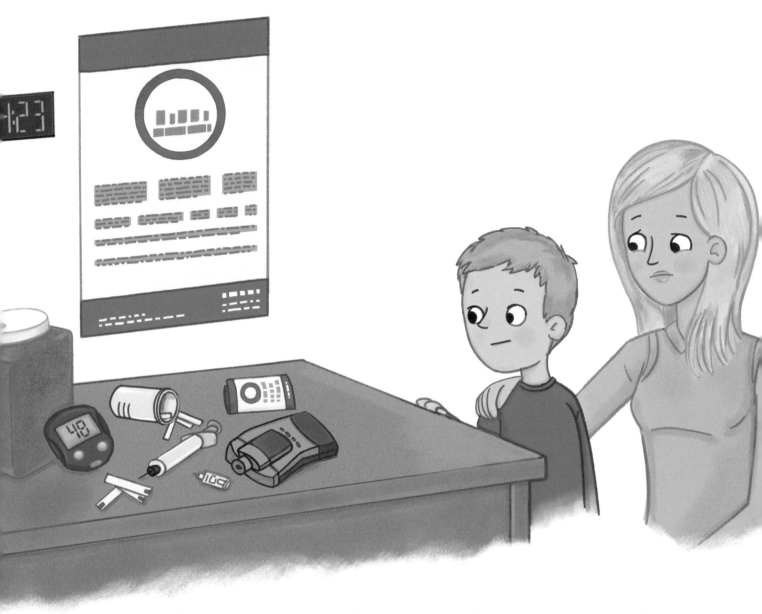

There are now things my brother must do.
My family will learn about diabetes too.

Food you eat gives you energy.
Glucose is sugar from the food, you see?

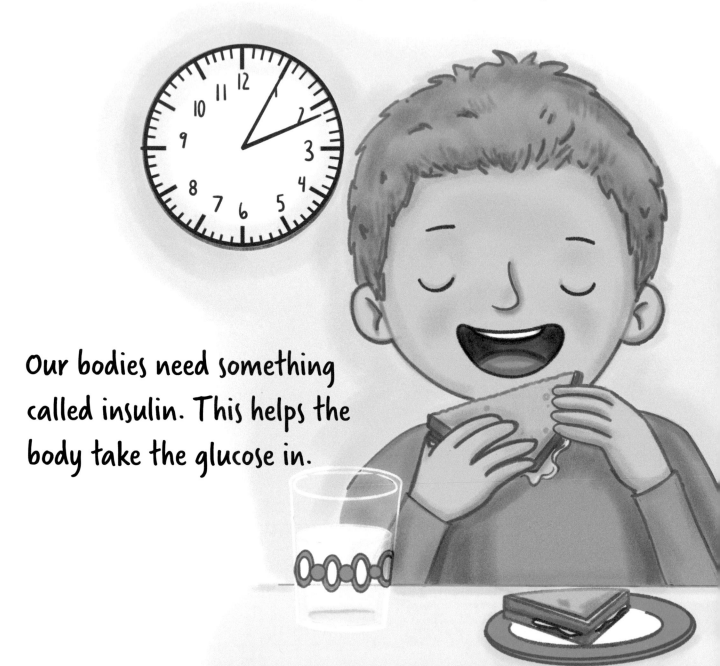

Our bodies need something
called insulin. This helps the
body take the glucose in.

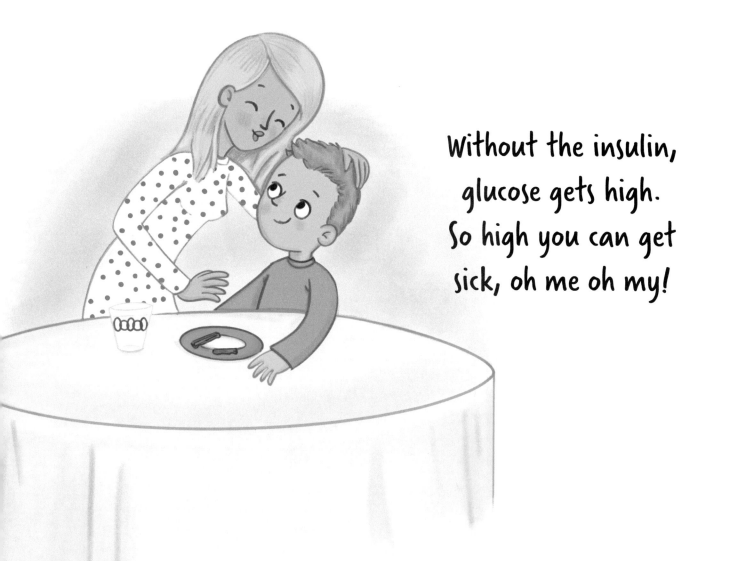

Without the insulin,
glucose gets high.
So high you can get
sick, oh me oh my!

Just one more time, let us go through this ...
But first, let mom give you a sweet kiss.

The body needs insulin.
It can't make enough.
The body needs help
and this next part's
tough ...

To keep the glucose from
making a jump, he will
need a shot or even a
pump.
Finger pokes with
needles had to begin.
His body had to start
getting more insulin.

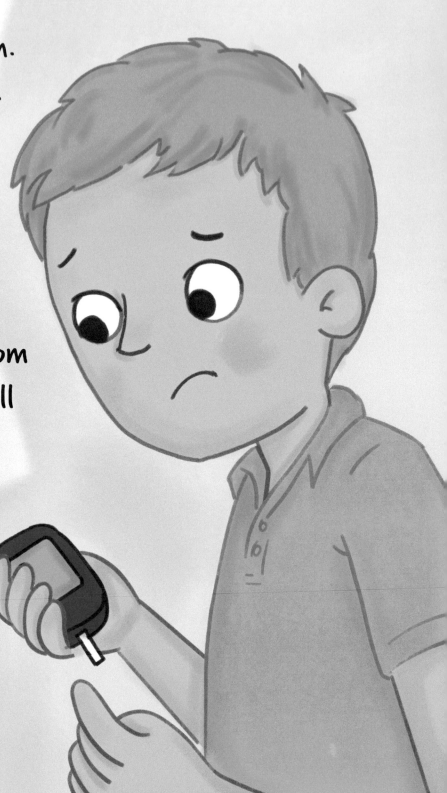

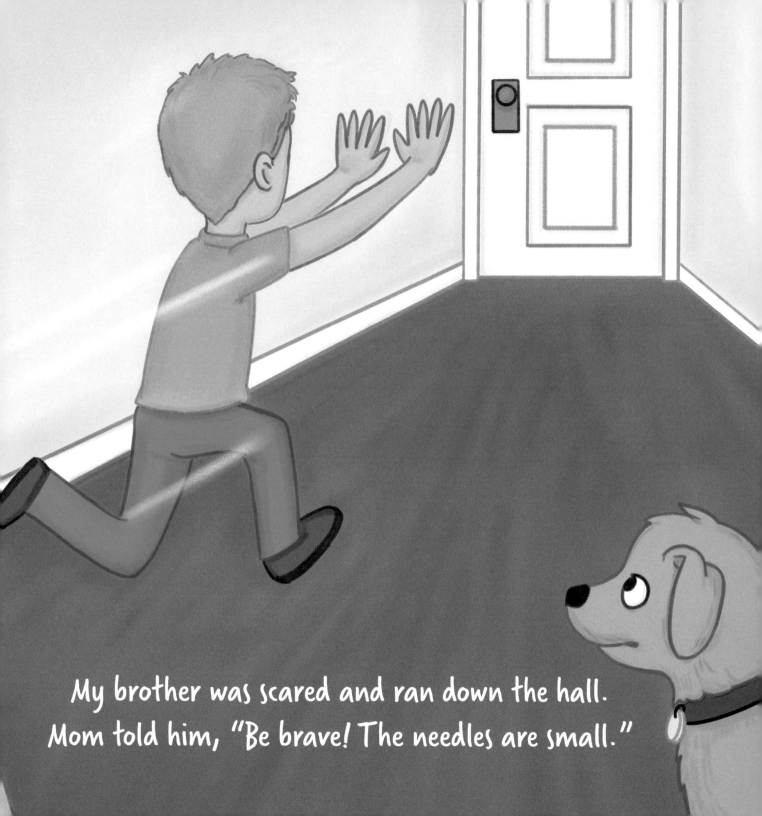

My brother was scared and ran down the hall.
Mom told him, "Be brave! The needles are small."

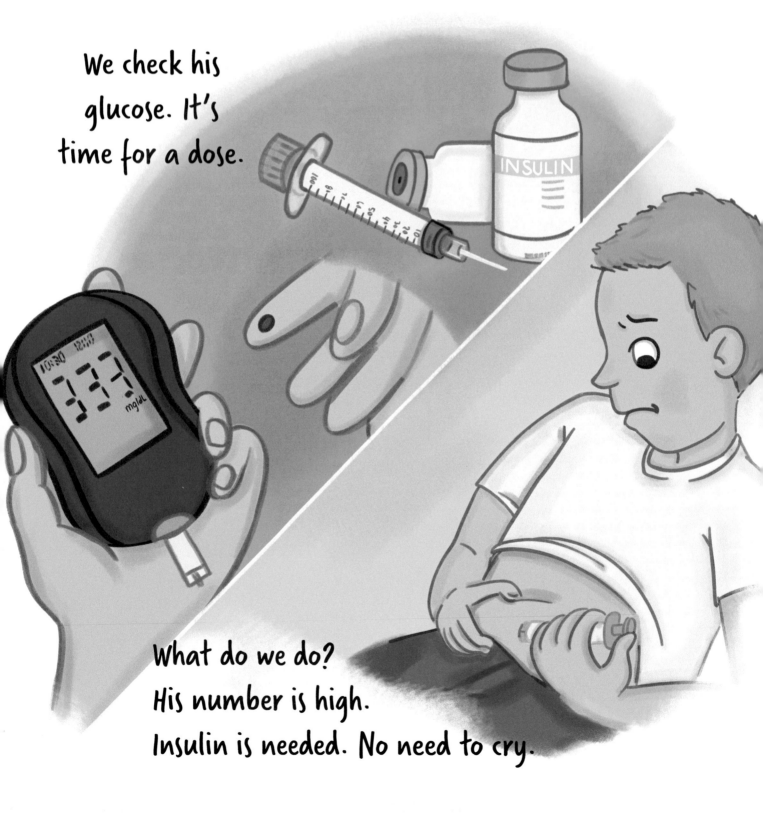

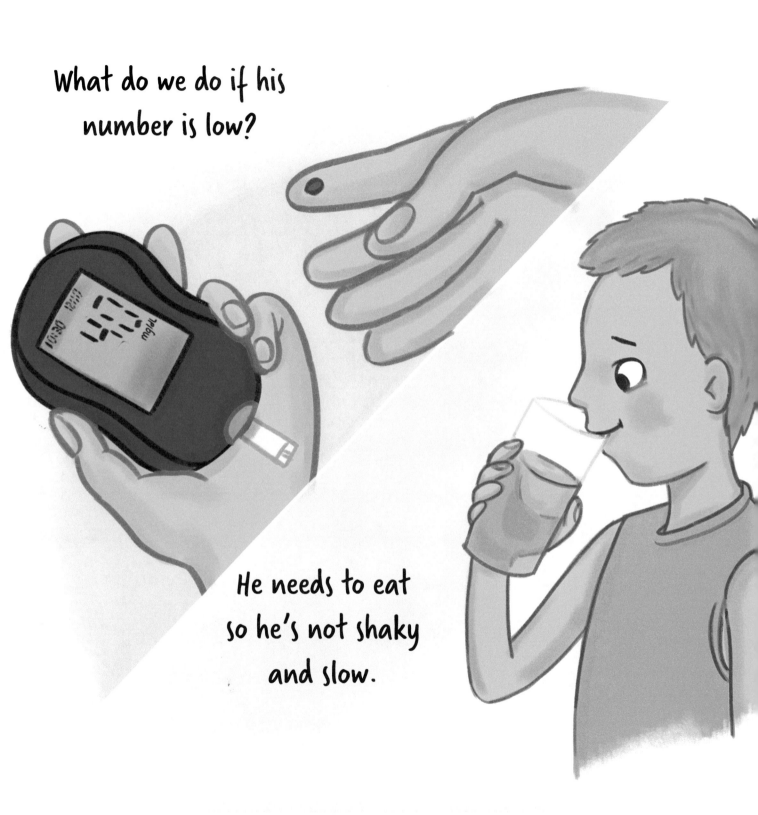

My brother now needs some rest and healing.
My mom wants to know how I am feeling.

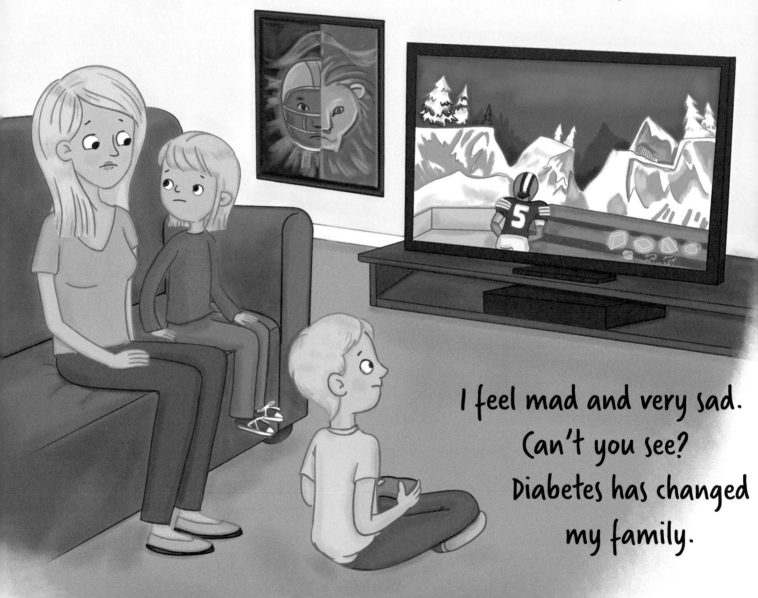

I feel mad and very sad.
Can't you see?
Diabetes has changed
my family.

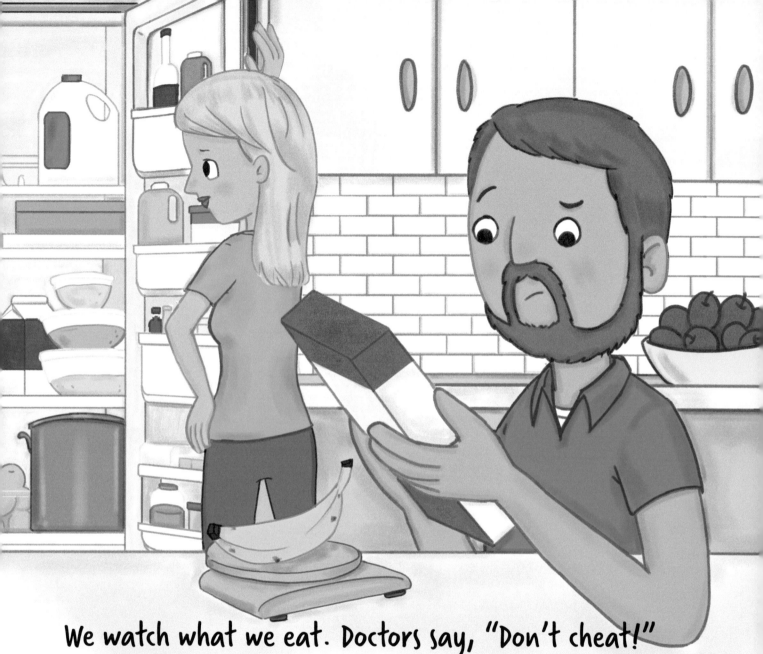

We watch what we eat. Doctors say, "Don't cheat!"
Yes to fruits and veggies. Limit sweet cakes.
Measuring each bite of food that he takes.

Brownies and pizza are now just a treat.
The family must focus on what we eat.

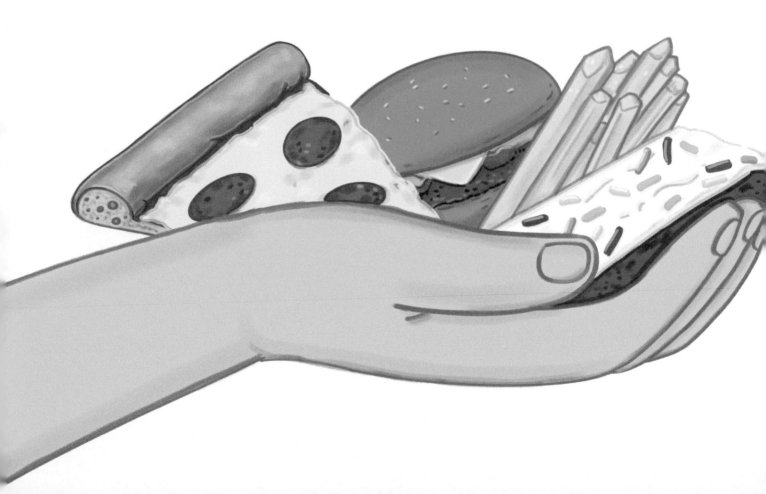

Food choices will need to be made.
Junk food for healthy food is the trade.

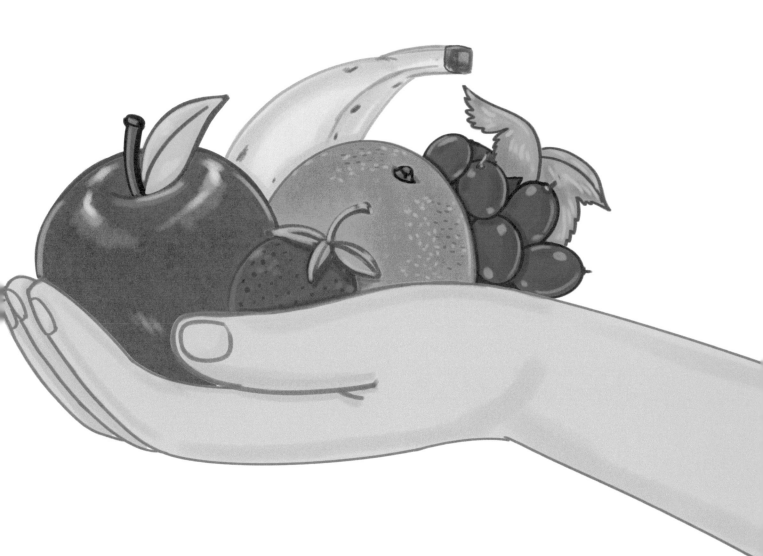

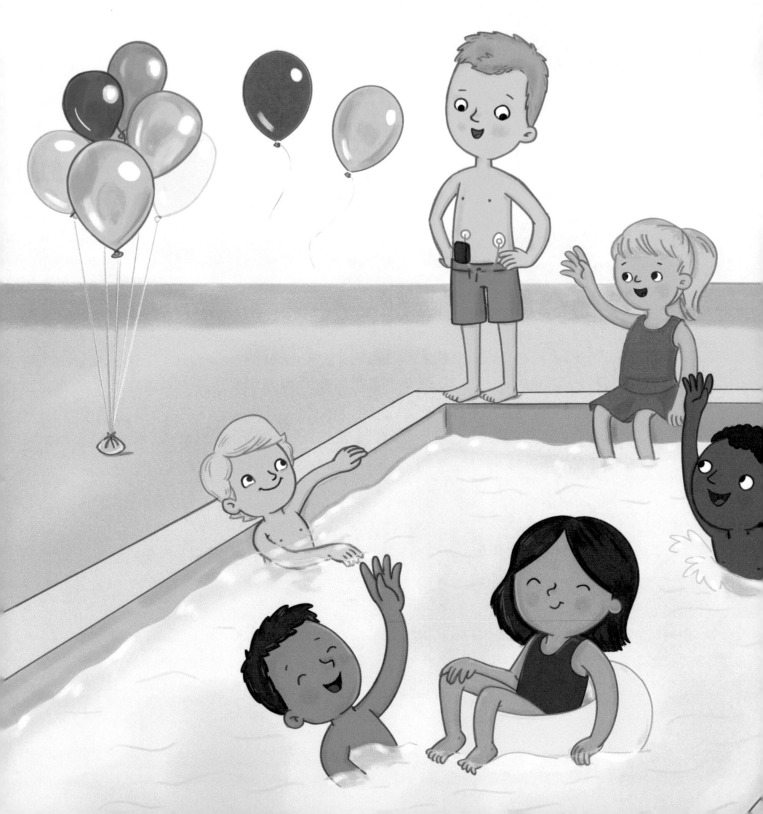

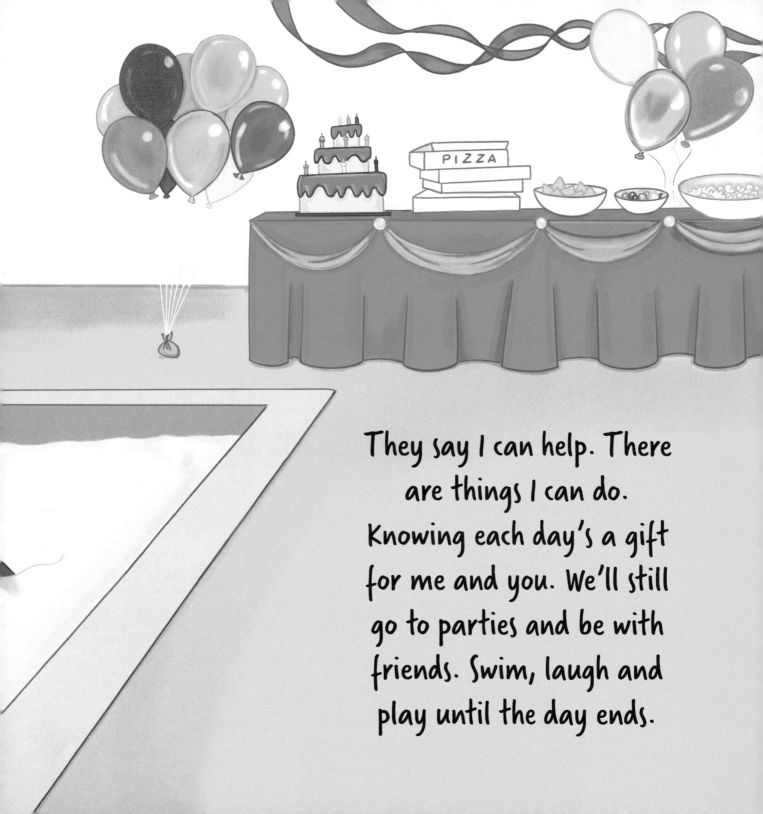

They say I can help. There are things I can do. Knowing each day's a gift for me and you. We'll still go to parties and be with friends. Swim, laugh and play until the day ends.

Nothing is sweeter than giving our love.
Let go and be happy. This they speak of…
Brothers and sisters can help lead the way. Find
the sweetness and joy in each new day.

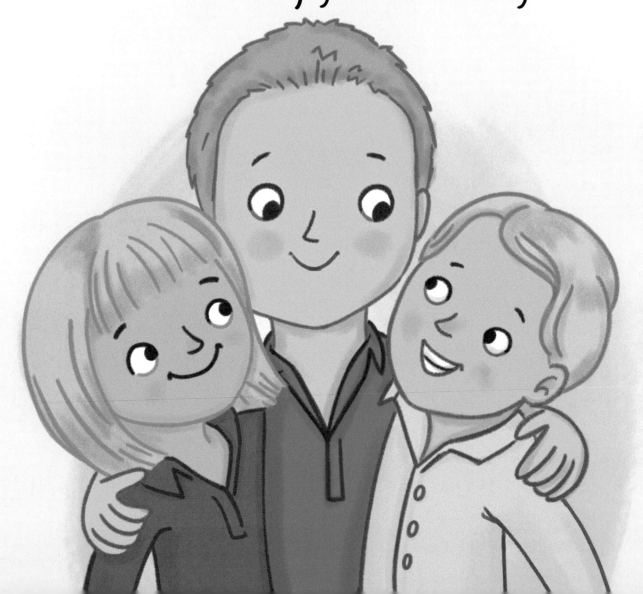

Dear Family,

Right now your head and hearts must be spinning. No doubt you're scared, overwhelmed, angry and are probably mourning the life you had or even thought you might have, particularly for your child. I want to tell you that these are very normal feelings and they will go away. My son, Dillon, was diagnosed with Type 1 diabetes three weeks after his 12th birthday. So many people told us that this is our "new normal". I even said it many times in the hopes of convincing myself and our family that it will eventually feel normal. The truth was, I didn't want to hear those words anymore. But, I am here to tell you that it does eventually feel normal. I promise. You and your beautiful family are now part of an exclusive club and I want to welcome you with open arms. I know it's not a club you would ever choose to be in but you are here and it is one of the strongest clubs there are. It is full of people who truly care and understand exactly what you guys are going through. We will pull you through, teach you, guide and support you. We get it and we will get you through it. As time goes by, you will begin to realize how strong this has made you and your family.

Type 1 diabetes isn't a diagnosis anyone wants, but there are so many positives that can come from it.....from strength, great people coming into your lives, and even health (yes Type 1s tend to be healthier than the average person) just to name a few. As devastating as a diagnosis this might be, it can also be not that terrible. As of this letter, I was in your shoes 7 years ago. I felt the same feelings you are feeling. I recently told my son that if I had one wish in life it would be to take Type 1 from him, even if it meant I would have to have it. His response was.... "then I wouldn't be who I am today". As a parent, that just made my heart melt. My son is one of the strongest, most organized, driven (and healthy) people I know and it is because he has Type 1. He is my hero. So, in closing, I want to tell you that you will be here too. You guys have got this!

Corinne

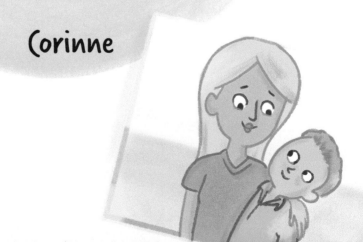

Printed in the United States
by Baker & Taylor Publisher Services